Honoring health and ditching diet:

...SECRETS TO BALANCED EATING

BY

WILDLY CHI

DISCLAIMER

TABLE OF CONTENTS

INTRODUCTION

Intuitive eating is a simple idea. It signifies that you make peace with all forms of cuisine. Unlike traditional diets restricting or banning certain foods, intuitive eating asks people to quit seeing food as "good" or "bad." instead, you listen to what your body tells you and consume what feels good.

This implies you eat anything you want, anytime. That's not the case. Experts say intuitive eating involves tapping into your body's ability to notify you when you're hungry or content.
A non-dieting strategy to modify your nutrition patterns is "intuitive eating."

Like the National Eating Disorders Association, intuitive eating is about respecting your body to make decisions regarding food that feel good for you without condemning yourself or the impact of diet culture.

"We're all born with the ability to know when to eat and when to stop eating, as well as what is pleasurable and satisfying," Rhonda explains.

"However, most of us start to become more disconnected and less trusting of our internal wisdom with the influence of family, friends, media, and diet culture."

After all, haven't we all given the keto diet, low-carb diet, eating small meals every 2 hours, and calorie restriction a fair go, only to cave into hunger and eat like lunatics when we lose control? And haven't we all felt terrible about consuming what we love too?

It means rejecting the so-called "diet rules" and eating the food that makes your body feel good—without the fear of judgment/guilt/adhering to the influence of the diet culture.

Intuitive eating is a strategy for health and wellness that enables you to tune into your body signals, ending the pattern of repetitive dieting and restoring your relationship with food.

In reality, if practiced appropriately, intuitive eating can give you a lot of benefits which are as follows:

Lower rate of emotional and disordered eating
Better body image
Boost self-esteem
Lower stress
Boost metabolism
Greater degrees of contentment and satisfaction

Intuitive eating may lead to a decrease in excessive eating disorders and eating for physical and psychological. INSIDE THIS BOOK, YOU LEARN THE SIMPLE STRATEGIES AND TIPS TO AVOID OVER EATING AND STICK TO INTUITIVE EATING; sit, relax, and stay tuned for these life-changing tips.

CHAPTER ONE

WHAT IS INTUITIVE EATING (IE)

Intuitive eating is a behavior or strategy that helps you to tune in to your body while enjoying varied foods without guilt or shame. It is popularly known as the "no diet" diet.

FACTS ABOUT INTUITIVE EATING

Intuitive eating is an excellent method to eliminate the vicious cycle of persistent dieting. It is true that most individuals who have been on dieting repeatedly will regain their weight. This is the famed yo-yo effect.

The harmful mindset around classifying things as "good" and evil and the guilt and shame that traditional diets generate around particular foods are associated with that.

Therefore, intuitive eating lets you experience freedom from food anxiety and appreciate your body's fundamental demands while making healthy food choices.

Guess what will happen: ultimately, you'll overindulge in those, leading to this sensation of shame and weight gain. Because of this, intuitive eating is more accurate in that it welcomes the act of savoring types of meals.

Admit it or not, this tendency is what helps you decide to balance and preserve a healthy weight in the long run.

GOAL ABOUT INTUITIVE EATING

The purpose of eating intuitively is to listen to your body and allow it to direct choices about when and how much to eat, rather than being affected by your surroundings, sentiments, or the norms given by diets. The concept is related to mindful eating; the two are often used interchangeably.

Mindful eating involves awareness of internal hunger and satiety indicators and making intentional meal choices. It emphasizes the necessity of paying attention to the emotional and physical experiences experienced when eating.

Despite many other diets, intuitive eating enables you to eat what you want - no food is a threat. While some may think that this could lead to adherents to the diet consuming more high-fat or high-sugar food, evidence reveals that this is not the case. Advocates of intuitive eating believe in eating.

The further you restrict yourself, the more predisposed you are to overeat later.

The notion of intuitive eating is straightforward and doesn't involve detailed dietary guidelines. But what does the evidence suggest?

No foods are off-limits with intuitive eating.

CHAPTER TWO

HOW TO PRACTICE INTUITIVE EATING

here's presenting the variables that you need to bear in mind if you want to give it a try:

Reject the diet mentality: From social media to publications to television, whatever it is that leads you to adopt restricted diets has got to be kicked out of your life forever. Because not only can they mislead you into following fad diets that might cause nutritional deficiencies in your body, but they can also make you feel incredibly terrible about not adhering to the claimed rules of dieting and ultimately damage your connection with food.

Honor your appetite: Starving yourself or neglecting your hunger will ultimately lead to food cravings and make you jump on food and binge eat when you finally lose control. Hence, eat when you're hungry and eat when you're full.

Occasional binge can't do you any harm, ladies. Make peace with food: Food is food. It could be better and better. We put these labels on them according to our delicious convenience. Indeed, a packet of chips isn't the healthiest option for you, but an occasional splurge in moderation will do you good. However, if you fight or restrict yourself, you can only end up binge-eating them in excess and feeling awful about it later.

That said, it's crucial to embrace healthy food as well. Certain foods make your body feel healthier and better. It would be best if you also kept in mind the nutritional worth of what you're eating. It's all about creating the appropriate balance between nutrients and taste.

Feel your fullness: Eating until you feel fed is vital, as dissatisfaction post a meal can encourage you to binge on snacks excessively and make you agitated.

Since your brain takes roughly 20 minutes to deliver signals of 'satisfaction' to your body, the ideal strategy is to chew your food properly, eat slowly, and pause between meals to decide if you're full. The objective is to listen to your body, you see?

Getting back in touch with the experience of eating and enjoying the food is crucial. So, be mindful of what you're eating and consume without interruptions while focusing on the meal's sight, smell, taste, and texture.

Discover the satisfaction factor: Another principle to remember here is that eating what is prescribed until you're full instead of eating what you feel can also contribute to discontent. Hence, you've got to honor your body's calling and eat what you're hankering for while considering the moderation issue.

Don't use food to cope with your emotions: Relying on an ice cream tub or a full-sized pizza in moments of happiness, despair, or confusion doesn't fit under intuitive eating, girls. That's nothing, just emotional eating.

Emotional hunger is utilizing food to make yourself feel better/to fulfill your emotional demands rather than fulfilling your hunger. One tends to consume based on feelings rather than the body's requirements.

Physical hunger is eating in reaction to the demand of the body to produce energy to carry out various physical activities. Your body starts to produce indications such as stomach grumbling, headache, and fatigue/exhaustion when it needs to get refueled.

Don't get confused between the two, and stop using food to cope with your emotions, okay?

Respect your body: Acceptance is crucial here. If you don't like your appearance and are overly critical of your body, you can never eat without feeling bad about it. A poor body image operates as a barrier to improving your relationship with food.

HOW TO EAT INTUITIVELY

Embracing intuitive eating all starts with the appropriate mindset. It's time to release the concerns about eating healthy and food in general. This is the key to a better living.

Reject diets: You may need more than rigid rules around eating to reduce weight over the long haul. If the diet is ineffective or you're unable to maintain your weight, it could happen.

Hunt for a higher, healthier diet and start all over again. When you restrict meals, your body's systems may not obtain the nutrients it needs to perform at its best. And for other people, frequent dieting could develop into an eating disorder.

Start with baby steps. Don't follow what others are doing. Just go with what works for you. Educate yourself on the importance of consuming a range of meals.

Intuitive eating is not a diet. It's something that you build slowly and fast repair. Instead, it is conduct that, over time, will influence you to build pleasant emotions around eating, food, and preparation.

Eat when you're hungry: Respect your body and give yourself the freedom to eat when it tells you you're starving. Consume various meals to ensure you obtain the nutrients you require. Please don't ignore your hunger feelings until they overpower you. Instead of picking foods that make you feel good, you're prone to consume everything you can obtain. You're also more inclined to overeat this way.

Stop classifying foods as "good" or "bad." Identify that each food has its particular value and nutrients. If you listen to your instincts, your body will accept your nutritious meals more significantly than others.

The same thing happens with exercising. Eating and exercise should not be a hardship or punishment for your body.

It would be best if you appreciated both as approaches to gaining excellent health.

Get into the habit of pampering and loving yourself more.

CHAPTER THREE
POSITIVE EFFECT ON THE BODY

In terms of weight loss, it has yet to be evident if intuitive eating is more beneficial than calorie restriction. Results from observational studies have indicated that persons who eat instinctively have a lower BMI (body mass index) than those who don't. However, since persons who restrict themselves may do so because they already have a high BMI, it is challenging to assess the actual effect intuitive eating has. Also, the outcomes from intervention trials with overweight or obese persons are not as noticeable.

For example, one analysis revealed that of the eight research they reviewed, just two found a reduction in weight through intuitive eating. In a more recent assessment, weight loss was seen in only eight out of 16 investigations. Yet weight loss was statistically substantial in only three of these eight.

Unlike previous diets, the primary objective of intuitive eating is not on fat loss but on addressing the reasons people eat. So, even if its efficiency as a strategy for weight loss is dubious, it could still bring benefits by fostering healthy eating habits.

This notion has been backed by research demonstrating intuitive eating might lead to a diminution in excessive eating symptoms and eating for physical and emotional reasons. Intuitive eating is also related to stronger positive body image, bodily satisfaction, improved emotional functioning, and higher self-esteem.

Finally, a recent study indicated that higher levels of intuitive feeding predicted reduced eating disorder symptoms, compared with calorie tracking and regular self-weighing. This contrasts with conventional restrictive dieting, which has been connected with a greater likelihood of eating problems, a risk that may be deeper for people who simultaneously experience sadness and low self-esteem symptoms.

LISTEN TO YOURSELF

One difficulty with intuitive eating is that it believes we can accurately identify how hungry or full we are. Research reveals that people better at perceiving internal sensations may also eat more instinctively. However, given there is evidence that people with eating disorders have difficulties identifying signals from inside their bodies, some people may struggle to respond to the intuitive eating strategy simply because they struggle to listen to their own bodies.

Also, while consuming based on internal sensations rather than exterior cues appears reasonable, there are more feasible solutions for many people. The time you eat is often out of your control, such as sticking to specified family mealtimes or designated periods at the workplace to have a lunch break. In contrast, in theory, eating when you're hungry seems perfect; it is only sometimes achievable.

Intuitive eating may be an efficient strategy to lose weight, but there is not enough evidence to demonstrate that it works better than standard, calorie-restrictive eating habits. But there are advantages to psychological health that consumed instinctively brings, suggesting that it is a much more healthful approach to eating.

It may not work for everyone, particularly individuals who struggle to perceive feelings in their own bodies. But at a time when everything in our surroundings is telling us what to eat and how much to consume, it may be worth spending time listening to your body to find out what you need.

CHAPTER FOUR

10 PRINCIPLES OF INTUITIVE EATING

What does intuitive eating mean?

Most of us were reared on three square meals a day - morning meal, lunch, and supper. And sometimes, if you are starving, you may eat a snack in between meals or top off your dinner with dessert.

While traditional mealtimes are acceptable, they only allow a few modifications. That's where intuitive eating comes in. Instead of being trapped into eating at specific times - even if you might not be hungry - intuitive eating is all about following your intuition and listening to your body's hunger cues for when to start eating and when to start.

How often have you been encouraged growing up to "eat everything on your plate; there are people worldwide that are starving!" Of course, we don't want to be wasteful, but our society has ingrained specific ways of thinking into our minds that disconnect us from our own internal wisdom of what works best for us and our bodies.

At its core, intuitive eating contains ten essential concepts that make this method what it is today:

1. Listen to your hunger

The first and most crucial aspect of intuitive eating is recognizing your hunger and honoring that hunger by eating. Your body is physiologically programmed to feel hungry when it requires sustenance. By rejecting that fundamental intuition, you are punishing your body and increasing your chance of overeating later.

2. Reject diet dogma

Many of our meal decisions are oriented around weight - whether we are attempting to lose weight or make sure we don't gain any more. It's no wonder we have such a massive diet culture in our society and a fascination with different eating methods, avoiding entire food groups, monitoring calories, and even eating disorders like anorexia and orthorexia.

Instead of getting caught up in the latest diet fads, intuitive eating redirects focus away from that group mentality and onto your own specific health path and goals. After all, in functional medicine, we realize that what works for one individual doesn't always work for the next. Intuitive eating embraces that concept in its totality and encourages you to eat what makes you feel good - not what a diet promises would make you feel good.

3. Discover true satisfaction

Are you genuinely paying attention to what you are eating? Food keeps us alive but is meant to be appreciated and relished. Why else are so many of life's milestones and celebrations centered around food? Intuitive eating realizes that food may be both a source of enjoyment and fuel. It also encourages us to slow down when eating, which helps us genuinely feel satisfied and realize when we are complete.

4. Make peace with food

Food is not the enemy. Instead, intuitive eating welcomes food as the potent, nourishing fuel that it is to generate energy for your body. Intuitive eating doesn't consider particular foods or food groupings as "bad" or "good." By acknowledging that food is supposed to fuel your body and bring personal satisfaction, you'll be permitting yourself to eat and will be able to make peace with every food that you put on your plate.

5. Find healthy coping techniques

Emotional eating is genuine for practically every one of us. Whether it be out of depression, anxiety, boredom, fear, or punishment, we might all have the urge to eat mindlessly, overeat, or not eat at all based on how we are feeling at the moment.

Intuitive eating urges you to pay attention to your emotional triggers and your response when it comes to food. Then you can begin to tackle the fundamental cause of why you turn to food to comfort your feelings and develop healthy coping techniques like movement, counseling, or mindfulness.

6. Find a movement you enjoy

We often stop eating due to the old "calories in, calories out" mentality. This can cause us to over-exercise in trying to justify the food we've consumed. However, once we have completely mastered intuitive eating, we'll quit punishing ourselves with activity because we have found peace with what we eat and how much we eat. Then, finding everyday exercise that you enjoy will become less about the results and more about wanting to celebrate and appreciate your body through movement.

7. Honor your health

There should be elegance and lightness to wellness. Intuitive eating knows that you don't become chronically ill or obese from one snack or meal. It's about the cumulative choices that you make over time. But when you learn to listen to your body, you'll give it precisely what it needs without overthinking it. And if you do consume something out of alignment with your body's needs? It's going to be okay. Give yourself grace and pick right back up where you left off!

8. Challenge the food police

Years of diet culture can have us believing some insane stringent lies about calories and particular foods. Instead of accepting these notions as "normal," challenge how they apply to you and throw anything that isn't helping you and your health goals out the window.

9. Love your body

As I constantly say, you can't cure a body you despise! Love the body you are in and honor it for all that it does for you. Understanding that only some people are going to look the same is the first step in appreciating yourself and using food to power your unique body composition.

10. Recognize what fullness feels like

Eating on the run or wiping our plates has yet to teach our bodies to detect when we are full. Intuitive eating wants us to slow down and learn what being full feels like so that we can eat just what our body desires - nothing more and nothing less.

THE BENEFITS OF INTUITIVE EATING

Intuitive eating is not simply another trendy wellness fad. Research has revealed that by following intuitive eating concepts, people showed:

Better cholesterol levels

Improved body image and self-esteem

Reduced stress

Increased satisfaction

Less eating disorders

Enhanced metabolism

Intuitive eating lets you spontaneously find foods that work for your body and which do not. It also goes further by helping you embrace your hunger and fullness signals, building a healthy connection with eating.

With natural eating, you are unlikely to discover it essential to measure or monitor calories and macros. Intuitive eating also fosters a mentality that is free from food deprivation and depression. Usually, our bodies tend to seek meals that we are deprived of. Demonizing food is a method of stating, "You don't have a choice to enjoy chocolate chip cupcakes cause you'll get overweight!"

CAN INTUITIVE EATING WORK FOR WEIGHT LOSS?

The encouraging aspect is that intuitive eating succeeds wonderfully in weight loss and fitness. The explanation is simple: this method becomes natural to you. Intuitive eating helps you get in shape.

Studies reveal that most people who learned to eat intuitively were able to build healthy connections to food, encountered less food anxiety, and obtained a healthy weight.

Your approach toward healthy eating positively transforms. It's a reality that the "dieting mindset" in which you continually watch calories, measure foods, and obsess over portion control only leads to eating disorders.

CHAPTER FIVE

WHAT IS DIETING

The term "diet" stems from the Greek word "diaita," literally meaning "manner of living." In the current discourse, dieting is connected with a quick-fix remedy for an overwhelming obesity crisis. Dieting entails restriction and reduction of enjoyable foods and drinks, and although having no advantages, the prevalent dieting attitude remains the standard.

Most diets fail most of the time. Repeated diet failure is a poor indicator of effective long-term weight loss. Chronic dieters regularly feel guilt, self-blame, irritation, anxiety and despair, difficulty concentrating, and weariness. Their self-esteem is reduced by recurrent emotions of failure connected to "making a mess my diet up again," leading to emotions of loss of influence over their food choices and, subsequently … life in general. Dieting may be particularly troublesome in teens, and it remains a crucial antecedent to disordered eating, with intermediate dieters being five times more likely to develop an eating bad habit than people who do not diet at all.

Diets indicate restriction. Psychologically, dietary constraints can lead to heightened responsiveness to food signals, increased desires and disinhibition, and overeating and binge eating. Biologically, dieting can lead to harmful changes in body composition, hormonal alterations, decreased bone density, menstrual irregularities, and lower resting energy expenditure.

DITCHING THE MINDSET OF DIETING

If one fact is actual, it's that there is no specific food that will keep you fit, and nor is there a single food that will get you fat.

All you have to do is make solid food decisions based on what feels organic to your body.

It has been historically presented that when you're liberated from food cravings, you make more nutritious choices and are at ease with food. Then, you naturally start reducing those unwanted pounds and lowering your waistline.

It's all about balance and the appropriate mindset.

To minimize dissatisfaction and body hate, you should emphasize eating in a style that works for you. There isn't a "one size fits all" strategy.

Everybody is unique. We all have distinct preferences and metabolism.
In reality, "dieting" without adequate counsel and supervision from a dietitian causes more damage than good. Believe me. That's why countless individuals experience the dreaded yo-yo effect.

So, instead of embracing the media cleanses, fasting regimens, and rapid solutions, you should begin learning how to tune in to your body. It is also crucial to discover how your body responds to your diet. You'll see better-lasting results.

IS INTUITIVE EATING DIET?

Intuitive eating is not a diet but a practice that will make you build pleasant feelings surrounding eating, food, and preparation.

DIFFERENCE BETWEEN INTUITIVE EATING AND DIETING

Dieting is a tight and structured eating style you must follow as you have picked it; it's typically following a set plan with its meal times, and calories, considering these variables. When it comes to traditional dieting, an individual is given a set of guidelines to follow to assist in losing weight. With intuitive eating, you learn to pay attention to what your body needs.

Intuitive eating is like toddlers; they focus on activities like play and only return when hungry. To describe it loosely, it involves no thought or planning, just connecting to your body and listening to it.

Intuitive eating implies you eat when you are hungry and stop precisely when you are about or full. You don't follow a set plan or watch calories and such.
It is about making peace with food. It's about learning how to listen to your body, how to acknowledge your hunger, and determining what to eat,

There are also no foods that are regarded as off-limits. However, that does not imply you should eat anything you want when you want. The secret is to identify when you're genuinely hungry.

Intuitive eating is a method everyone can utilize. However, you should consult your physician for specific medical conditions like diabetes or high blood pressure.

DOES INTUITIVE EATING BETTER THAN COUNTING CALORIES?

If you've been dieting or calculating calories, not seeing results, feeling out of control, or spending too much time worrying about food, give intuitive eating a shot. You'll wind up balancing your diet out a lot better. Take a nibble of the cookie, have a glass of wine on the weekend, and if you are taken away during the week, that's alright! It's not the end of the world, we promise. If portion management is your problem, establish a meal program; stop tracking calories, start feeding yourself, and feel the difference.

WHY DIETING IS NOT THE BEST WAY TO EAT

Effects of dieting: Aggressive dieting decreases the basal metabolic rate, meaning one consumes less energy when resting, resulting in much reduced daily requirements to preserve the obtained weight when the diet is complete. Returning to typical eating patterns at this decreased base metabolic rate leads to widely witnessed post-dieting weight gain. Biologically, dieting is viewed as damaging, and physiology readjusts attempting to return to the initial weight even after years following the first fast weight reduction. A recent study investigating 14 participants in the "Biggest Loser" contest showed they shed, on a typical basis, 128 pounds, and their baseline resting rates of metabolism reduced from 2,607 +/- 649 kilocalories/ single day to 1,996 +/- 358 kcal/day at the conclusion of the 30 weeks event. Those that shed the most significant weight showed the largest decreases in their metabolic rate. Six years after the program, only one of the 14 participants weighed less than they did during the competition; five contestants recovered almost all of or more than the weight they lost, yet despite the weight increase, their metabolic rates stayed modest, with an average of 1,903 +/- 466 kcal/day. Equal to their weights, the contenders were burning a mean of ~500 fewer kilocalories a whole day than should be anticipated of persons their size leading to continuous weight gain over the years. Metabolic adaptation connected to fast weight reduction remained over time, demonstrating a proportionate but imperfect response to concurrent attempts to lower body weight from its designated "set point."

Dieting promotes food as "good" or "bad" as a reward or punishment and creates food obsessions. It does not teach good eating habits and rarely focuses on the nutritional content of foods and the advantages of regulated eating. Unsatisfied hunger promotes mood swings and the danger of overeating. Restricting meals and even drinking enough water can lead to dehydration and other issues, such as constipation. Dieting and persistent hunger worsen dysfunctional habits like smoking cigarettes or drinking alcohol.

Complex concepts like health and wellness cannot be reduced to one isolated figure what body mass index (BMI) is. Significance and value cannot be determined by weight. A dieting mindset tempts us into the "thinking If I am thin- I will be pleased" or "If I am not, thin-I am a failure" manner that thinks but only delivers a short-term false solution with long-term damaging bodily and emotional implications. Focusing on sustainable long-term solutions for establishing controlled eating habits with a range of food choices without excessive limits will make a comprehensive diet and maintaining a healthy weight a natural part of our "manner of living."

Dieting can impact your metabolism, your capacity to sense hunger and fullness and make you feel worried, guilty, or humiliated about eating

THE HEALTHIEST WAY TO EAT

Eating a variety of healthful meals is the most unique approach to make sure you satisfy your micronutrient demands. To make healthy selections, search for nutrient-dense foods. These are foods high in micronutrients yet low in calories. Nutrient-dense choices include fruits and vegetables, healthy grains, lean protein, and low-fat dairy.

CHAPTER SIX

WHAT INTUITIVE EATING LOOKS LIKE

Intuitive eaters choose foods based on hunger, fullness, and enjoyment instead of long-held eating norms, constraints, or other external considerations. They trust their body to tell them when, what, and exactly how much. It's a non-judgment technique that removes guilt and shame around eating.

LOVING YOURSELF MORE THAN YOUR BODY AND MINDSET

Remember that your sentiments are valid. You're staying in touch with reality. You know yourself better than anybody else, so be your greatest advocate.

Focus on self-love and self-compassion rather than attempting to persuade others to ... It's time to calm down and allow your body and mind to relax.

Start by selecting a pleasurable activity. · Focus on eating healthily. · Keep affirming notes around. · Decorate your desk. And be joyful

CONCLUSION

Extant research reveals multiple and persistent connections between intuitive eating, reduced BMI, and greater psychological well-being. Additional studies can add to the range and depth of these results. The essay finishes with several suggestions for further investigation.

Rhonda employs a "weight-unbiased" methodology to assist people in modifying their life activities and food connections rather than focusing on being in shape. According to Rhonda, many individuals come to her for help reducing weight. Instead, she helps them understand why they need to be in shape, what their prior experiences with overindulging have shown them, and alternate methods by which they may accomplish their goals without changing their body size. In any event, I would determine how it impacts them, whether to reduce their glucose or pulse or give them more energy. We would also explore what they might undertake to "get fitter to be better." We want to focus on shadows and moving motions rather than the quantity of the scale."

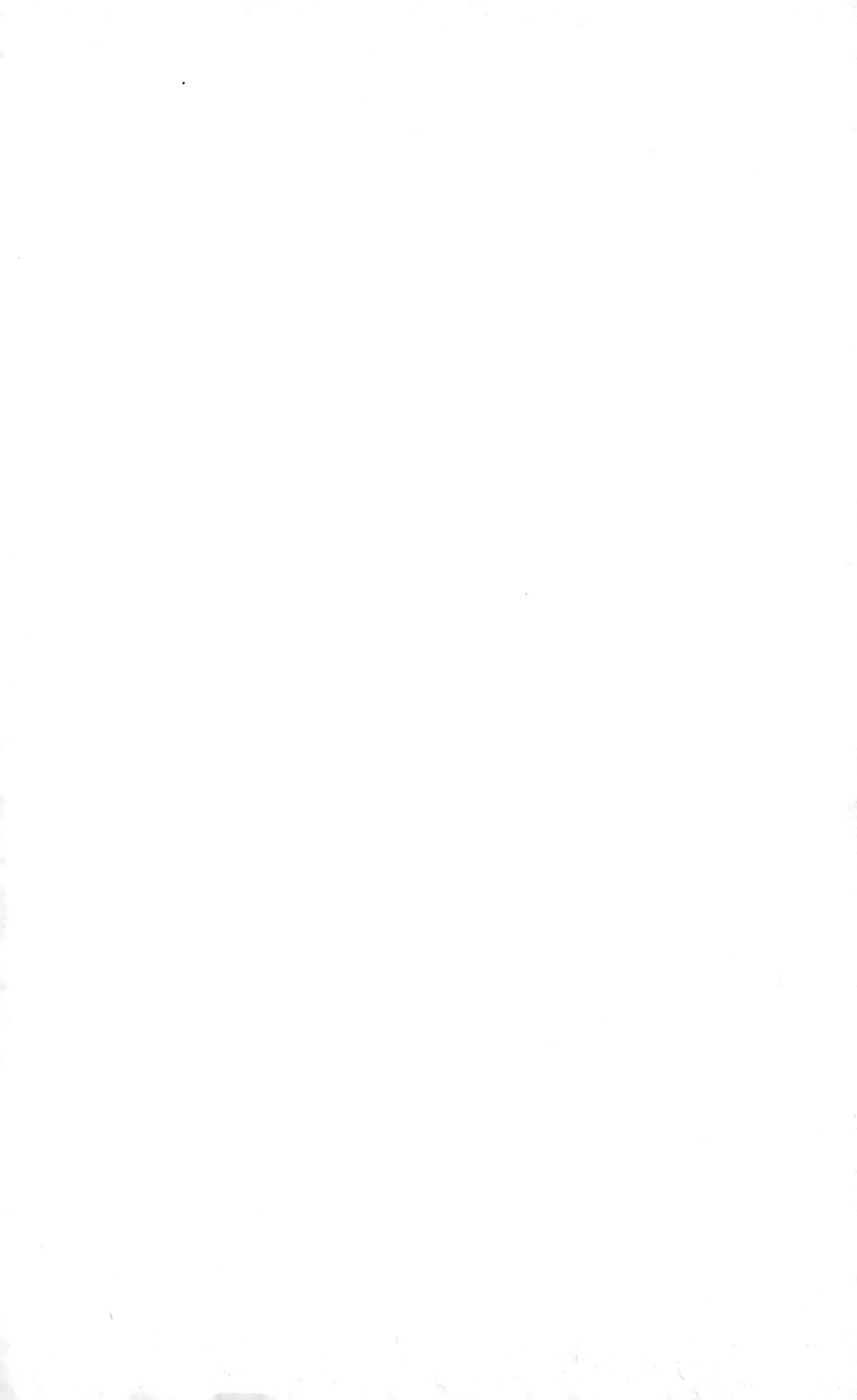

www.ingramcontent.com/pod-product-compliance
Lightning Source LLC
Chambersburg PA
CBHW071044260726
48661CB00007B/3158